# CONTENTS

# INTRODUCTION

### History and Cultural Significance

The practice of postpartum confinement, known as "sitting the month" or "zuo yue zi," has deep roots in Chinese culture, dating back thousands of years. It is a period during which a new mother takes extensive rest, adheres to a specific diet, and follows certain lifestyle restrictions to ensure optimal recovery and long-term health. The tradition is based on the belief that childbirth depletes a woman's body of essential energy and nutrients, making her vulnerable to illnesses and imbalances. By observing confinement, it is believed that a woman can restore her health and regain her strength more effectively.

### The Principles of Traditional Chinese Medicine in Confinement

Traditional Chinese Medicine (TCM) plays a pivotal role in confinement practices. TCM principles emphasize the balance of yin and yang, the vital forces that govern health and wellbeing. After childbirth, a woman's body is considered to be in a state of yin (cold) deficiency. To counteract this, confinement practices focus on replenishing yang (heat) through dietary choices and lifestyle adjustments. This involves consuming warming foods, avoiding cold environments, and promoting blood circulation to support healing and recovery.

### Benefits of Confinement for New Mothers

Confinement practices offer numerous benefits for new mothers, both physically and emotionally. These include:

- **Physical Healing**: The body undergoes significant

changes during pregnancy and childbirth. Confinement helps in healing the uterus, reducing postpartum bleeding, and promoting the healing of any tears or incisions.

- **Energy Restoration**: The specialized diet and rest help restore energy levels depleted during labor and delivery.

- **Improved Lactation**: Certain foods and herbs consumed during confinement can boost milk production and improve its quality, supporting successful breastfeeding.

- **Hormonal Balance**: The practice aids in stabilizing hormone levels, reducing the risk of postpartum depression and mood swings.

- **Enhanced Immunity**: The nutrient-rich diet strengthens the immune system, protecting the mother from infections and illnesses.

## Modern Adaptations and Practices

While traditional confinement practices remain popular, modern adaptations have emerged to accommodate contemporary lifestyles. These include:

- **Professional Confinement Centers**: Specialized facilities where new mothers receive comprehensive care, including meals, medical check-ups, and support from trained professionals.

- **Customized Confinement Packages**: Home delivery of confinement meals tailored to individual dietary needs and preferences.

- **Flexible Guidelines**: Allowing for more moderate restrictions on activities and diet to suit individual comfort levels and health conditions.

## The Importance of Nutrition During Confinement

## Healing and Recovery Post-Childbirth

Nutrition is crucial for postpartum recovery. A diet rich in protein, vitamins, and minerals supports the repair of tissues and the healing of wounds. Foods like chicken, fish, and eggs provide essential amino acids needed for muscle and tissue repair. Iron-rich foods help replenish blood loss and prevent anemia.

## Enhancing Milk Production

Certain foods are believed to enhance milk production and improve its quality. Ingredients like papaya, fish, and various herbal soups are traditionally consumed to boost lactation. Adequate hydration and a balanced intake of nutrients are also vital for maintaining a healthy milk supply.

## Restoring Energy Levels

Childbirth is an exhausting process, and new mothers often experience fatigue. A nutrient-dense diet helps restore energy levels. Complex carbohydrates, healthy fats, and proteins provide sustained energy, while foods like red dates and longan are used in TCM for their energy-boosting properties.

## Balancing Hormones

Hormonal fluctuations after childbirth can affect a mother's mood and physical health. A balanced diet rich in omega-3 fatty acids, vitamins, and minerals can help stabilize hormone levels. Foods like fatty fish, nuts, seeds, and leafy greens are beneficial for hormonal balance.

## Strengthening the Immune System

A strong immune system is essential for new mothers to ward off infections and recover quickly. Nutrient-rich foods, including fruits, vegetables, and whole grains, provide antioxidants and other immune-boosting compounds. Herbal soups and teas are also used in TCM to enhance immunity and overall health.

By understanding and embracing these principles, new mothers can navigate the postpartum period with greater ease and confidence, ensuring a healthy start for both themselves and their newborns.

# CHAPTER 1: PROTEIN-RICH FOODS

**Importance of Protein for Healing and Recovery**

Protein plays a crucial role in the postpartum recovery process. After childbirth, a woman's body undergoes significant physical stress and requires adequate nutrients to heal and regain strength. Protein is an essential nutrient that supports the body's repair mechanisms and promotes overall recovery.

Proteins are made up of amino acids, which are the building blocks of cells and tissues. Consuming sufficient protein helps to:

- **Repair Damaged Tissues**: Childbirth can cause tears, incisions, and other forms of tissue damage. Protein intake supports the healing of these tissues, ensuring a faster and more effective recovery.

- **Replenish Blood Supply**: Proteins are essential for the production of hemoglobin, a component of red blood cells that carries oxygen throughout the body. This is particularly important after childbirth, as blood loss can occur during delivery.

- **Boost Immune Function**: Proteins are vital for the production of antibodies and other immune cells that protect the body against infections. A strong immune system is crucial for new mothers, who may be more susceptible to illnesses during the postpartum period.

## Enhancing Muscle and Tissue Repair

Postpartum recovery involves the restoration of muscle strength and the repair of connective tissues. Protein-rich foods provide the necessary amino acids for these processes:

- **Muscle Repair and Growth**: Pregnancy and childbirth can strain the muscles, particularly those in the pelvic region and abdomen. Consuming adequate protein supports muscle repair and growth, helping new mothers regain their physical strength.

- **Collagen Production**: Collagen is a protein that provides structure to the skin, tendons, and ligaments. It plays a vital role in the healing of perineal tears or cesarean section incisions. Foods rich in protein help boost collagen production, promoting faster wound healing.

- **Maintaining Skin Elasticity**: Protein contributes to the maintenance of skin elasticity, which can be affected by the stretching that occurs during pregnancy. Adequate protein intake helps improve skin health and reduces the risk of postpartum skin issues.

By incorporating protein-rich foods into their diet, new mothers can support their body's natural healing processes and ensure a smoother postpartum recovery. In the following sections, we will explore a variety of delicious and nutritious recipes that are rich in protein and designed to enhance healing and recovery.

## Recipes

### 1. Ginger Chicken Soup

**Ingredients:**

- 1 whole chicken, cut into pieces
- 2-inch piece of ginger, sliced
- 4 cups chicken broth

- 2 tablespoons sesame oil
- Salt to taste

## Instructions:

1. Heat sesame oil in a pot and sauté the ginger slices until fragrant.
2. Add the chicken pieces and cook until they are lightly browned.
3. Pour in the chicken broth and bring to a boil.
4. Reduce heat and simmer for 1 hour, or until the chicken is tender.
5. Season with salt to taste and serve hot.

## 2. Black Chicken Herbal Soup

### Ingredients:

- 1 black chicken, cut into pieces
- 1 small piece of ginseng
- 6 dried red dates
- 2 slices of dang gui (Chinese angelica root)
- 6 cups water
- Salt to taste

## Instructions:

1. Rinse the black chicken pieces and set aside.
2. In a pot, combine the chicken, ginseng, red dates, dang gui, and water.
3. Bring to a boil, then reduce heat and simmer for 2 hours.
4. Season with salt to taste and serve hot.

## 3. Steamed Cod with Ginger and Soy Sauce

### Ingredients:

- 2 cod fillets

- 1-inch piece of ginger, julienned
- 2 tablespoons soy sauce
- 1 tablespoon sesame oil
- 1 tablespoon rice wine
- 2 green onions, chopped

**Instructions:**

1. Place the cod fillets on a steaming plate and top with ginger julienne.
2. In a small bowl, mix soy sauce, sesame oil, and rice wine.
3. Pour the mixture over the fish.
4. Steam the fish over boiling water for 10-12 minutes, or until cooked through.
5. Garnish with chopped green onions and serve hot.

## 4. Braised Pork with Black Vinegar

**Ingredients:**

- 500g pork belly, cut into chunks
- 1 cup black vinegar
- 1/2 cup soy sauce
- 1/4 cup brown sugar
- 2 cloves garlic, minced
- 2-inch piece of ginger, sliced
- 1 cup water

**Instructions:**

1. In a pot, combine black vinegar, soy sauce, brown sugar, garlic, ginger, and water.
2. Add the pork belly chunks and bring to a boil.
3. Reduce heat and simmer for 1.5 to 2 hours, or until the pork is tender and the sauce has thickened.

4.  Serve hot with rice.

## 5. Steamed Egg Custard

**Ingredients:**

- 4 eggs
- 1 cup chicken broth
- 1/2 teaspoon salt
- 1 tablespoon sesame oil
- Chopped green onions for garnish

**Instructions:**

1.  Beat the eggs in a bowl and mix in the chicken broth and salt.
2.  Strain the mixture to remove any bubbles.
3.  Pour the egg mixture into small heatproof bowls or ramekins.
4.  Steam over low heat for 15-20 minutes, or until the custard is set.
5.  Drizzle with sesame oil and garnish with chopped green onions before serving.

# CHAPTER 2: IRON-RICH FOODS

**Importance of Iron for Blood Replenishment**

Iron is a crucial nutrient for new mothers, especially after childbirth, when the body needs to replenish lost blood and support overall recovery. Iron plays a vital role in the production of hemoglobin, the protein in red blood cells that carries oxygen to tissues and organs. Adequate iron intake ensures that the body can produce enough healthy red blood cells to replace those lost during delivery, promoting faster healing and recovery.

**Preventing Postpartum Anemia**

Postpartum anemia is a common condition that can occur due to significant blood loss during childbirth. Symptoms of anemia include fatigue, weakness, dizziness, and shortness of breath. Consuming iron-rich foods helps prevent anemia by boosting the body's iron stores and supporting the production of red blood cells. This is particularly important for new mothers, as anemia can impede the recovery process and affect their ability to care for their newborn.

In the following sections, we will explore a variety of delicious and nutritious recipes that are rich in iron and designed to enhance blood replenishment and prevent postpartum anemia.

**Recipes**

**1. Braised Pork Liver with Ginger**

**Ingredients:**

- 500g pork liver, sliced
- 2 tablespoons sesame oil
- 2-inch piece of ginger, julienned
- 2 cloves garlic, minced
- 2 tablespoons soy sauce
- 1 tablespoon oyster sauce
- 1/2 cup water
- Chopped green onions for garnish

**Instructions:**

1. Rinse the pork liver slices under cold water and pat dry.
2. Heat sesame oil in a pan and sauté the ginger and garlic until fragrant.
3. Add the pork liver slices and cook until browned on both sides.
4. Add soy sauce, oyster sauce, and water to the pan.
5. Bring to a boil, then reduce heat and simmer for 10-15 minutes, or until the liver is cooked through and the sauce has thickened.
6. Garnish with chopped green onions and serve hot.

## 2. Spinach and Red Dates Soup

**Ingredients:**

- 2 cups fresh spinach leaves
- 10 dried red dates, pitted
- 1 piece of dried tangerine peel (optional)
- 4 cups chicken or vegetable broth
- Salt to taste

**Instructions:**

1. Rinse the spinach leaves and set aside.

2. In a pot, bring the chicken or vegetable broth to a boil.

3. Add the dried red dates and tangerine peel (if using) to the pot.

4. Reduce heat and simmer for 20 minutes.

5. Add the spinach leaves and cook for an additional 5 minutes, or until the spinach is wilted.

6. Season with salt to taste and serve hot.

## 3. Beef and Spinach Stir-Fry

### Ingredients:

- 300g beef tenderloin, thinly sliced
- 2 tablespoons soy sauce
- 1 tablespoon oyster sauce
- 2 cloves garlic, minced
- 2 cups fresh spinach leaves
- 1 tablespoon sesame oil
- 1 tablespoon cornstarch
- 1/4 cup water
- Salt and pepper to taste

### Instructions:

1. In a bowl, marinate the beef slices with soy sauce, oyster sauce, and cornstarch. Set aside for 10 minutes.

2. Heat sesame oil in a pan and sauté the garlic until fragrant.

3. Add the marinated beef slices and stir-fry until browned.

4. Add the spinach leaves and stir-fry until wilted.

5. Pour in the water and cook for an additional 2-3 minutes, or until the sauce has thickened.

6. Season with salt and pepper to taste and serve hot.

## 4. Chicken Liver Pate

**Ingredients:**

- 500g chicken livers, cleaned and trimmed
- 1 small onion, finely chopped
- 2 cloves garlic, minced
- 1/4 cup brandy or cognac (optional)
- 1/2 cup unsalted butter, softened
- 1 tablespoon olive oil
- 1 teaspoon fresh thyme leaves
- Salt and pepper to taste

**Instructions:**

1. Heat olive oil in a pan and sauté the onion and garlic until softened.
2. Add the chicken livers and cook until browned on the outside but still slightly pink inside.
3. Pour in the brandy or cognac (if using) and cook until the liquid has evaporated.
4. Transfer the mixture to a food processor and blend until smooth.
5. Add the softened butter and thyme leaves, and blend until well combined.
6. Season with salt and pepper to taste.
7. Transfer the pate to a serving dish and chill in the refrigerator for at least 1 hour before serving.

## 5. Sesame Oil Chicken with Red Dates

**Ingredients:**

- 1 whole chicken, cut into pieces

- 2 tablespoons sesame oil
- 10 dried red dates, pitted
- 1-inch piece of ginger, sliced
- 2 cups chicken broth
- Salt to taste

**Instructions:**

1. Heat sesame oil in a pot and sauté the ginger slices until fragrant.
2. Add the chicken pieces and cook until browned on all sides.
3. Add the dried red dates and chicken broth to the pot.
4. Bring to a boil, then reduce heat and simmer for 45 minutes to 1 hour, or until the chicken is tender.
5. Season with salt to taste and serve hot.

# CHAPTER 3: WARMING FOODS

**The Role of Warming Foods in Traditional Chinese Medicine**

In Traditional Chinese Medicine (TCM), the concept of balancing yin and yang is essential for maintaining health. After childbirth, a woman's body is considered to be in a state of yin (cold) deficiency, which can lead to various health issues if not addressed properly. To restore balance and promote recovery, TCM emphasizes the consumption of yang (warming) foods during the postpartum period. These warming foods help to replenish the body's energy, improve blood circulation, and enhance overall vitality.

**Promoting Circulation and Digestion**

Warming foods play a significant role in promoting circulation and digestion, which are crucial for postpartum recovery. Improved circulation helps to deliver essential nutrients and oxygen to tissues, supporting healing and reducing the risk of complications. Enhanced digestion ensures that the body can efficiently absorb the nutrients needed for recovery. Warming foods also help to expel cold from the body, reducing the likelihood of discomfort and promoting overall well-being.

In the following sections, we will explore a variety of delicious and nutritious recipes that are designed to warm the body, promote circulation, and improve digestion.

**Recipes**

## 1. Ginger and Vinegar Pig's Trotters

**Ingredients:**

- 2 pig's trotters, cleaned and cut into pieces
- 1 cup black vinegar
- 1/2 cup rice vinegar
- 2-inch piece of ginger, sliced
- 4 cloves garlic, minced
- 2 tablespoons brown sugar
- 4 cups water
- Salt to taste

**Instructions:**

1. In a large pot, combine the black vinegar, rice vinegar, ginger, garlic, brown sugar, and water. Bring to a boil.
2. Add the pig's trotters to the pot and bring back to a boil.
3. Reduce heat and simmer for 2-3 hours, or until the trotters are tender and the sauce has thickened.
4. Season with salt to taste and serve hot.

## 2. Turmeric Chicken Soup

**Ingredients:**

- 1 whole chicken, cut into pieces
- 1 tablespoon turmeric powder
- 2-inch piece of ginger, sliced
- 4 cloves garlic, minced
- 4 cups chicken broth
- 2 tablespoons olive oil
- Salt and pepper to taste

**Instructions:**

1. Heat olive oil in a pot and sauté the ginger and garlic until fragrant.

2. Add the chicken pieces and cook until browned on all sides.

3. Add the turmeric powder and stir to coat the chicken evenly.

4. Pour in the chicken broth and bring to a boil.

5. Reduce heat and simmer for 1 hour, or until the chicken is tender.

6. Season with salt and pepper to taste and serve hot.

## 3. Sesame Oil Fried Rice

**Ingredients:**

- 2 cups cooked rice (preferably day-old)
- 2 tablespoons sesame oil
- 1-inch piece of ginger, julienned
- 2 cloves garlic, minced
- 2 eggs, beaten
- 1 cup mixed vegetables (carrots, peas, corn)
- 2 tablespoons soy sauce
- Chopped green onions for garnish

**Instructions:**

1. Heat sesame oil in a large pan or wok and sauté the ginger and garlic until fragrant.

2. Add the beaten eggs and scramble until cooked.

3. Add the mixed vegetables and stir-fry for a few minutes.

4. Add the cooked rice and soy sauce, and stir-fry until everything is well combined and heated through.

5. Garnish with chopped green onions and serve hot.

## 4. Black Vinegar Pork Trotters

**Ingredients:**

- 2 pig's trotters, cleaned and cut into pieces
- 1 cup black vinegar
- 1/2 cup rice vinegar
- 1/4 cup brown sugar
- 2-inch piece of ginger, sliced
- 4 cups water
- Salt to taste

**Instructions:**

1. In a large pot, combine the black vinegar, rice vinegar, brown sugar, ginger, and water. Bring to a boil.
2. Add the pig's trotters to the pot and bring back to a boil.
3. Reduce heat and simmer for 2-3 hours, or until the trotters are tender and the sauce has thickened.
4. Season with salt to taste and serve hot.

## 5. Ginger Tea with Red Dates

**Ingredients:**

- 2-inch piece of ginger, sliced
- 10 dried red dates, pitted
- 4 cups water
- 2 tablespoons brown sugar (optional)

**Instructions:**

1. In a pot, combine the ginger slices, red dates, and water. Bring to a boil.
2. Reduce heat and simmer for 30 minutes.
3. If desired, add brown sugar to taste and stir until dissolved.

4.  Strain the tea into cups and serve hot.

These recipes are designed to warm the body, promote circulation, and support digestion, making them ideal for the postpartum period. By incorporating these warming foods into their diet, new mothers can enhance their recovery and ensure a healthy start for themselves and their newborns.

# CHAPTER 4: SOUPS AND BROTHS

**The Nutritional Benefits of Soups and Broths**

Soups and broths are a staple in postpartum diets due to their numerous health benefits. They are not only comforting and easy to consume but also packed with essential nutrients that support healing and recovery. The slow cooking process used to prepare soups and broths helps to extract maximum nutrients from the ingredients, making them highly nutritious.

**Easy Digestion and Hydration**

Soups and broths are easily digestible, which is particularly important for new mothers whose digestive systems may be weakened post-delivery. The warm liquid helps to soothe the digestive tract and can improve nutrient absorption. Additionally, soups and broths contribute to hydration, an essential factor for recovery and breastfeeding.

In the following sections, we will explore a variety of delicious and nutritious recipes for soups and broths that are designed to support postpartum recovery.

**Recipes**

**1. Chicken and Papaya Soup**

**Ingredients:**

- 1 whole chicken, cut into pieces
- 1 unripe papaya, peeled, seeded, and cut into chunks

- 2-inch piece of ginger, sliced
- 4 cups chicken broth
- 2 tablespoons sesame oil
- Salt to taste

**Instructions:**

1. Heat sesame oil in a pot and sauté the ginger slices until fragrant.
2. Add the chicken pieces and cook until browned on all sides.
3. Add the papaya chunks and chicken broth to the pot.
4. Bring to a boil, then reduce heat and simmer for 1 hour, or until the chicken is tender.
5. Season with salt to taste and serve hot.

## 2. Fish and Papaya Soup

**Ingredients:**

- 2 white fish fillets (such as cod or tilapia)
- 1 unripe papaya, peeled, seeded, and cut into chunks
- 2-inch piece of ginger, sliced
- 4 cups fish or chicken broth
- 2 tablespoons sesame oil
- Salt to taste

**Instructions:**

1. Heat sesame oil in a pot and sauté the ginger slices until fragrant.
2. Add the fish fillets and cook until lightly browned.
3. Add the papaya chunks and broth to the pot.
4. Bring to a boil, then reduce heat and simmer for 30 minutes, or until the fish is cooked and the papaya is

tender.

5. Season with salt to taste and serve hot.

## 3. Bone Broth with Goji Berries

**Ingredients:**

- 2 pounds beef or chicken bones
- 2-inch piece of ginger, sliced
- 1/2 cup goji berries
- 1 onion, quartered
- 4 cloves garlic, peeled
- 8 cups water
- Salt to taste

**Instructions:**

1. In a large pot, combine the bones, ginger, onion, garlic, and water. Bring to a boil.
2. Reduce heat and simmer for at least 4 hours, skimming off any foam that rises to the surface.
3. Add the goji berries during the last 30 minutes of cooking.
4. Strain the broth through a fine mesh sieve.
5. Season with salt to taste and serve hot.

## 4. Herbal Chicken Soup

**Ingredients:**

- 1 whole chicken, cut into pieces
- 2 pieces of dried astragalus root
- 2 pieces of dried dang gui (Chinese angelica root)
- 4 dried red dates, pitted
- 2-inch piece of ginger, sliced

- 4 cups chicken broth
- Salt to taste

**Instructions:**

1. Rinse the chicken pieces and set aside.
2. In a pot, combine the chicken, astragalus root, dang gui, red dates, ginger, and chicken broth.
3. Bring to a boil, then reduce heat and simmer for 2 hours.
4. Remove the herbs and ginger slices before serving.
5. Season with salt to taste and serve hot.

## 5. Pork Rib and Lotus Root Soup

**Ingredients:**

- 500g pork ribs, cut into pieces
- 1 lotus root, peeled and sliced
- 4 dried red dates, pitted
- 2 slices of ginger
- 4 cups chicken or pork broth
- Salt to taste

**Instructions:**

1. Blanch the pork ribs in boiling water for a few minutes to remove impurities. Drain and set aside.
2. In a pot, combine the pork ribs, lotus root slices, red dates, ginger, and broth.
3. Bring to a boil, then reduce heat and simmer for 1.5 to 2 hours, or until the ribs are tender and the lotus root is soft.
4. Season with salt to taste and serve hot.

These soups and broths are not only nourishing but also easy to digest and hydrating, making them perfect for new mothers during the postpartum period. By incorporating these recipes into their diet, new mothers can support their recovery and ensure they are getting the nutrients they need to heal and thrive.

# CHAPTER 5: WHOLE GRAINS AND CARBOHYDRATES

### Importance of Carbohydrates for Energy

Carbohydrates are a primary source of energy for the body, making them essential for postpartum recovery. New mothers need ample energy to heal, produce breast milk, and care for their newborns. Whole grains and other complex carbohydrates provide sustained energy by releasing glucose slowly into the bloodstream. This steady supply of energy helps to prevent fatigue and supports overall well-being during the demanding postpartum period.

### Maintaining Blood Sugar Levels

Maintaining stable blood sugar levels is crucial for new mothers, as it helps to avoid energy crashes and mood swings. Whole grains and other complex carbohydrates have a low glycemic index, meaning they do not cause rapid spikes and drops in blood sugar levels. Including these foods in a postpartum diet ensures a more balanced and consistent energy supply, aiding in physical recovery and emotional stability.

In the following sections, we will explore a variety of delicious and nutritious recipes that are rich in whole grains and carbohydrates, designed to provide energy and maintain stable blood sugar levels.

### Recipes

## 1. Confinement Rice with Herbs

**Ingredients:**

- 1 cup jasmine rice
- 2 tablespoons sesame oil
- 2 slices of ginger
- 1 tablespoon dried goji berries
- 2 cups chicken broth
- 1/4 cup chopped fresh herbs (such as parsley, cilantro, or basil)
- Salt to taste

**Instructions:**

1. Rinse the jasmine rice under cold water and drain.
2. Heat sesame oil in a pot and sauté the ginger slices until fragrant.
3. Add the rice and goji berries, stirring to coat with the oil.
4. Pour in the chicken broth and bring to a boil.
5. Reduce heat, cover, and simmer for 15-20 minutes, or until the rice is cooked and the liquid is absorbed.
6. Remove from heat and let it sit for 5 minutes.
7. Fluff the rice with a fork, remove the ginger slices, and stir in the chopped herbs.
8. Season with salt to taste and serve hot.

## 2. Brown Rice Porridge with Red Dates

**Ingredients:**

- 1 cup brown rice
- 8 dried red dates, pitted and chopped
- 4 cups water
- 1 tablespoon brown sugar (optional)

- 1/2 teaspoon salt

**Instructions:**

1. Rinse the brown rice under cold water and drain.

2. In a pot, combine the brown rice, red dates, and water.

3. Bring to a boil, then reduce heat and simmer for 45 minutes to 1 hour, or until the rice is soft and the mixture has a porridge-like consistency.

4. Stir in the brown sugar (if using) and salt.

5. Serve hot.

### 3. Oatmeal with Dried Longan and Goji Berries

**Ingredients:**

- 1 cup rolled oats

- 4 cups water or milk (or a combination of both)

- 1/4 cup dried longan

- 1/4 cup dried goji berries

- 1 tablespoon honey or maple syrup (optional)

- 1/2 teaspoon cinnamon (optional)

**Instructions:**

1. In a pot, combine the rolled oats, water or milk, dried longan, and dried goji berries.

2. Bring to a boil, then reduce heat and simmer for 10-15 minutes, or until the oats are soft and the mixture has thickened.

3. Stir in the honey or maple syrup and cinnamon (if using).

4. Serve hot.

### 4. Sweet Potato Rice

**Ingredients:**

- 1 cup jasmine or basmati rice
- 1 medium sweet potato, peeled and diced
- 2 tablespoons sesame oil
- 2 cups water or chicken broth
- Salt to taste

**Instructions:**

1. Rinse the rice under cold water and drain.
2. Heat sesame oil in a pot and sauté the diced sweet potato for a few minutes.
3. Add the rice and stir to coat with the oil.
4. Pour in the water or chicken broth and bring to a boil.
5. Reduce heat, cover, and simmer for 15-20 minutes, or until the rice and sweet potato are cooked and the liquid is absorbed.
6. Remove from heat and let it sit for 5 minutes.
7. Fluff the rice with a fork, season with salt to taste, and serve hot.

## 5. Millet Porridge

**Ingredients:**

- 1 cup millet
- 4 cups water or chicken broth
- 1/4 cup dried goji berries
- 1 tablespoon honey or brown sugar (optional)
- 1/2 teaspoon salt

**Instructions:**

1. Rinse the millet under cold water and drain.
2. In a pot, combine the millet, water or chicken broth, and dried goji berries.

3. Bring to a boil, then reduce heat and simmer for 30-40 minutes, or until the millet is soft and the mixture has a porridge-like consistency.

4. Stir in the honey or brown sugar (if using) and salt.

5. Serve hot.

These recipes are designed to provide sustained energy and maintain stable blood sugar levels, making them ideal for new mothers during the postpartum period. By incorporating these whole grains and carbohydrates into their diet, new mothers can support their recovery and ensure they have the energy needed to care for themselves and their newborns.

# CHAPTER 6: VEGETABLES

**Nutritional Benefits of Vegetables**

Vegetables are a cornerstone of a healthy diet, providing essential vitamins, minerals, fiber, and antioxidants. These nutrients support various bodily functions, promote healing, and enhance overall well-being. For new mothers, a diet rich in vegetables can aid in postpartum recovery by boosting the immune system, improving digestion, and providing sustained energy.

**Importance of Cooked Vegetables During Confinement**

In Traditional Chinese Medicine, cooked vegetables are preferred over raw ones during the confinement period. Cooking vegetables makes them easier to digest, which is crucial for new mothers as their digestive systems may be weakened post-delivery. Cooked vegetables also help to warm the body and prevent the introduction of cold, which is believed to be harmful during the postpartum period. Incorporating a variety of cooked vegetables into the diet ensures that new mothers receive the necessary nutrients for optimal recovery.

In the following sections, we will explore a variety of delicious and nutritious recipes that feature cooked vegetables, designed to support postpartum recovery.

**Recipes**

**1. Stir-Fried Spinach with Garlic**

**Ingredients:**

- 2 cups fresh spinach leaves
- 3 cloves garlic, minced
- 2 tablespoons sesame oil
- 1 tablespoon soy sauce
- Salt to taste

**Instructions:**

1. Heat sesame oil in a pan over medium heat.
2. Add the minced garlic and sauté until fragrant.
3. Add the spinach leaves and stir-fry until wilted.
4. Add the soy sauce and stir to combine.
5. Season with salt to taste and serve hot.

## 2. Braised Kale with Ginger

**Ingredients:**

- 1 bunch kale, stems removed and leaves chopped
- 2-inch piece of ginger, sliced
- 2 tablespoons olive oil
- 1 cup vegetable or chicken broth
- Salt and pepper to taste

**Instructions:**

1. Heat olive oil in a pot over medium heat.
2. Add the sliced ginger and sauté until fragrant.
3. Add the chopped kale and stir to coat with the oil.
4. Pour in the broth and bring to a boil.
5. Reduce heat and simmer for 15-20 minutes, or until the kale is tender.
6. Season with salt and pepper to taste and serve hot.

## 3. Carrot and Ginger Soup

**Ingredients:**

- 4 large carrots, peeled and chopped
- 1 onion, chopped
- 2-inch piece of ginger, sliced
- 4 cups vegetable broth
- 2 tablespoons olive oil
- Salt and pepper to taste

**Instructions:**

1. Heat olive oil in a pot over medium heat.
2. Add the chopped onion and sliced ginger, and sauté until the onion is translucent.
3. Add the chopped carrots and stir to combine.
4. Pour in the vegetable broth and bring to a boil.
5. Reduce heat and simmer for 20-25 minutes, or until the carrots are tender.
6. Blend the soup with an immersion blender until smooth.
7. Season with salt and pepper to taste and serve hot.

**4. Sweet Potato and Carrot Mash**

**Ingredients:**

- 2 large sweet potatoes, peeled and chopped
- 2 large carrots, peeled and chopped
- 2 tablespoons butter or ghee
- 1/4 cup milk or chicken broth
- Salt and pepper to taste

**Instructions:**

1. Bring a large pot of water to a boil.

2. Add the chopped sweet potatoes and carrots, and cook until tender, about 15-20 minutes.

3. Drain and return the vegetables to the pot.

4. Add the butter or ghee and milk or chicken broth.

5. Mash the vegetables until smooth and creamy.

6. Season with salt and pepper to taste and serve hot.

## 5. Steamed Bok Choy with Sesame Oil

### Ingredients:

- 4 heads baby bok choy, halved lengthwise
- 2 tablespoons sesame oil
- 1 tablespoon soy sauce
- 1 tablespoon toasted sesame seeds
- Salt to taste

### Instructions:

1. Steam the bok choy halves until tender, about 5-7 minutes.

2. Transfer the bok choy to a serving dish.

3. Drizzle with sesame oil and soy sauce.

4. Sprinkle with toasted sesame seeds.

5. Season with salt to taste and serve hot.

These vegetable recipes are designed to provide essential nutrients, support digestion, and promote overall well-being, making them ideal for new mothers during the postpartum period. By incorporating these cooked vegetables into their diet, new mothers can enhance their recovery and ensure they are getting the nutrients they need to heal and thrive.

# CHAPTER 7:
# HERBAL TEAS

**Benefits of Herbal Teas for Postpartum Recovery**

Herbal teas have been used for centuries to support health and well-being, and they play a particularly important role in postpartum recovery. Rich in antioxidants, vitamins, and minerals, herbal teas can help to boost the immune system, promote healing, and support overall health. They are also known for their soothing properties, which can help new mothers to relax and manage stress.

**Hydration and Relaxation**

Staying hydrated is crucial for new mothers, especially those who are breastfeeding. Herbal teas provide a delicious and beneficial way to ensure adequate hydration. Many herbal teas also have calming effects, which can help to reduce anxiety, promote better sleep, and support emotional well-being during the postpartum period.

In the following sections, we will explore a variety of herbal tea recipes that are designed to support postpartum recovery by providing hydration, relaxation, and a range of health benefits.

**Recipes**

**1. Red Date and Longan Tea**

**Ingredients:**

- 10 dried red dates, pitted

- 10 dried longans
- 4 cups water
- 1 tablespoon honey (optional)

**Instructions:**

1. Rinse the red dates and dried longans under cold water.
2. In a pot, combine the red dates, longans, and water.
3. Bring to a boil, then reduce heat and simmer for 30 minutes.
4. Strain the tea into cups.
5. Stir in honey if desired and serve hot.

## 2. Ginger and Brown Sugar Tea

**Ingredients:**

- 2-inch piece of ginger, sliced
- 4 cups water
- 2 tablespoons brown sugar (or to taste)

**Instructions:**

1. In a pot, combine the sliced ginger and water.
2. Bring to a boil, then reduce heat and simmer for 20 minutes.
3. Strain the tea into cups.
4. Stir in brown sugar until dissolved and serve hot.

## 3. Goji Berry and Red Date Tea

**Ingredients:**

- 1/4 cup dried goji berries
- 10 dried red dates, pitted
- 4 cups water

**Instructions:**

1. Rinse the goji berries and red dates under cold water.
2. In a pot, combine the goji berries, red dates, and water.
3. Bring to a boil, then reduce heat and simmer for 20 minutes.
4. Strain the tea into cups and serve hot.

## 4. Longan and Ginger Tea

**Ingredients:**

- 10 dried longans
- 2-inch piece of ginger, sliced
- 4 cups water
- 1 tablespoon honey (optional)

**Instructions:**

1. Rinse the dried longans under cold water.
2. In a pot, combine the longans, sliced ginger, and water.
3. Bring to a boil, then reduce heat and simmer for 25-30 minutes.
4. Strain the tea into cups.
5. Stir in honey if desired and serve hot.

## 5. Chinese Wolfberry Tea

**Ingredients:**

- 1/4 cup dried Chinese wolfberries (goji berries)
- 4 cups water
- 1 tablespoon honey (optional)

**Instructions:**

1. Rinse the Chinese wolfberries under cold water.
2. In a pot, combine the wolfberries and water.
3. Bring to a boil, then reduce heat and simmer for 20 minutes.

4. Strain the tea into cups.

5. Stir in honey if desired and serve hot.

These herbal tea recipes are designed to provide hydration, relaxation, and a range of health benefits, making them perfect for new mothers during the postpartum period. By incorporating these soothing and nutritious teas into their daily routine, new mothers can enhance their recovery and ensure they are taking care of both their physical and emotional well-being.

# CHAPTER 8: DAIRY ALTERNATIVES

**Nutritional Benefits of Dairy**

Dairy products are an excellent source of essential nutrients such as calcium, protein, vitamin D, and various B vitamins. These nutrients play a vital role in supporting bone health, muscle function, and overall recovery during the postpartum period. Calcium is particularly important for new mothers as it helps to replenish bone density and support the production of breast milk. The protein found in dairy aids in tissue repair and muscle recovery, making it a valuable addition to the diet.

**Suitable Dairy Alternatives**

For those who are lactose intolerant, vegan, or simply prefer not to consume dairy, there are plenty of nutritious alternatives available. Dairy alternatives, such as almond milk, soy milk, and coconut milk, can provide many of the same benefits as traditional dairy products. These alternatives are often fortified with calcium, vitamin D, and other essential nutrients to ensure they support postpartum recovery effectively.

In the following sections, we will explore a variety of delicious and nutritious recipes that include both dairy and suitable dairy alternatives, ensuring all new mothers can enjoy the benefits of these important nutrients.

**Recipes**

**1. Milk and Red Date Smoothie**

**Ingredients:**

- 1 cup milk (or plant-based milk)
- 5 dried red dates, pitted and soaked in warm water
- 1 banana
- 1 tablespoon honey
- 1/2 teaspoon vanilla extract

**Instructions:**

1. Drain the soaked red dates.
2. In a blender, combine milk, red dates, banana, honey, and vanilla extract.
3. Blend until smooth.
4. Pour into a glass and serve immediately.

## 2. Yogurt with Goji Berries and Nuts

**Ingredients:**

- 1 cup plain yogurt (or plant-based yogurt)
- 2 tablespoons dried goji berries
- 2 tablespoons mixed nuts (such as almonds, walnuts, or cashews)
- 1 tablespoon honey (optional)

**Instructions:**

1. In a bowl, combine yogurt, goji berries, and mixed nuts.
2. Stir well to mix.
3. Drizzle with honey if desired.
4. Serve immediately.

## 3. Cheese and Herb Omelette

**Ingredients:**

- 2 eggs

- 2 tablespoons milk (or plant-based milk)
- 1/4 cup grated cheese (or dairy-free cheese)
- 1/4 cup chopped fresh herbs (such as parsley, chives, or dill)
- Salt and pepper to taste
- 1 tablespoon butter or oil

**Instructions:**

1. In a bowl, beat the eggs with milk, salt, and pepper.
2. Heat butter or oil in a non-stick pan over medium heat.
3. Pour the egg mixture into the pan and cook until it starts to set.
4. Sprinkle grated cheese and chopped herbs on one half of the omelette.
5. Fold the other half over the filling and cook until the cheese is melted and the eggs are fully set.
6. Serve hot.

## 4. Almond Milk Porridge

**Ingredients:**

- 1 cup almond milk
- 1/2 cup rolled oats
- 1 tablespoon almond butter
- 1 tablespoon honey or maple syrup
- 1/4 cup fresh or dried fruits (such as berries, banana slices, or raisins)
- Pinch of cinnamon

**Instructions:**

1. In a pot, combine almond milk and rolled oats.
2. Bring to a boil, then reduce heat and simmer for 5-7

minutes, stirring occasionally.

3. Stir in almond butter, honey or maple syrup, and cinnamon.

4. Cook for another 1-2 minutes until thickened.

5. Serve in bowls topped with fresh or dried fruits.

## 5. Chia Seed Pudding with Longan

**Ingredients:**

- 1/4 cup chia seeds
- 1 cup coconut milk (or other plant-based milk)
- 1 tablespoon honey or maple syrup
- 1 teaspoon vanilla extract
- 1/4 cup dried longan

**Instructions:**

1. In a bowl, combine chia seeds, coconut milk, honey or maple syrup, and vanilla extract.

2. Stir well to mix.

3. Cover and refrigerate for at least 4 hours or overnight, until the mixture has thickened.

4. Stir again before serving and top with dried longan.

**These recipes provide a variety of delicious ways to incorporate dairy and dairy alternatives into a postpartum diet, offering essential nutrients to support bone health, muscle recovery, and overall well-being. By including these nutrient-rich options in their daily meals, new mothers can enhance their recovery and ensure they are getting the necessary nutrients for optimal health during the postpartum period.**

# CHAPTER 9: NUTS AND SEEDS

**Nutritional Benefits of Nuts and Seeds**

Nuts and seeds are nutritional powerhouses, packed with essential vitamins, minerals, healthy fats, protein, and fiber. They provide a wide range of nutrients such as vitamin E, magnesium, zinc, and omega-3 fatty acids, all of which are crucial for postpartum recovery. These nutrients support various bodily functions, including immune system health, skin health, and cardiovascular health.

**Importance for Energy and Lactation**

Nuts and seeds are excellent sources of energy due to their high content of healthy fats and protein. This makes them an ideal snack for new mothers who need sustained energy to care for their newborns. Additionally, certain nuts and seeds, like almonds and sesame seeds, are believed to promote lactation and improve the quality of breast milk. Including these foods in a postpartum diet can help new mothers maintain their energy levels and support successful breastfeeding.

In the following sections, we will explore a variety of delicious and nutritious recipes that incorporate nuts and seeds, designed to support postpartum recovery and enhance energy and lactation.

**Recipes**

**1. Almond and Sesame Seed Soup**

**Ingredients:**

- 1/2 cup almonds
- 2 tablespoons white sesame seeds
- 4 cups water
- 2 tablespoons honey (optional)
- Pinch of salt

## Instructions:

1. Soak the almonds in water for at least 4 hours or overnight.
2. Rinse the soaked almonds and sesame seeds.
3. In a blender, combine the almonds, sesame seeds, and water. Blend until smooth.
4. Pour the mixture into a pot and bring to a boil.
5. Reduce heat and simmer for 10-15 minutes.
6. Add honey and salt, stirring to combine.
7. Serve hot.

## 2. Walnut and Red Date Congee

## Ingredients:

- 1/2 cup walnuts
- 10 dried red dates, pitted and chopped
- 1 cup rice
- 6 cups water
- 1 tablespoon brown sugar (optional)
- Pinch of salt

## Instructions:

1. Rinse the rice under cold water and drain.
2. In a pot, combine the rice, water, chopped red dates, and walnuts.

3. Bring to a boil, then reduce heat and simmer for 1 hour, stirring occasionally.

4. Add brown sugar and salt, stirring to combine.

5. Serve hot.

### 3. Sunflower Seed and Goji Berry Snack Bars

**Ingredients:**

- 1 cup sunflower seeds
- 1/2 cup dried goji berries
- 1 cup rolled oats
- 1/2 cup honey or maple syrup
- 1/4 cup almond butter
- 1 teaspoon vanilla extract
- Pinch of salt

**Instructions:**

1. Preheat the oven to 350°F (175°C) and line a baking dish with parchment paper.

2. In a large bowl, combine sunflower seeds, goji berries, and rolled oats.

3. In a small pot, heat honey or maple syrup, almond butter, vanilla extract, and salt over low heat until smooth.

4. Pour the wet mixture over the dry ingredients and mix until well combined.

5. Press the mixture into the prepared baking dish.

6. Bake for 20-25 minutes or until golden brown.

7. Allow to cool completely before cutting into bars.

### 4. Sesame Seed and Black Bean Soup

**Ingredients:**

- 1/2 cup black beans
- 2 tablespoons black sesame seeds
- 1 onion, chopped
- 2 cloves garlic, minced
- 4 cups vegetable broth
- 2 tablespoons olive oil
- Salt and pepper to taste

## Instructions:

1. Soak the black beans in water overnight.
2. Rinse and drain the beans.
3. Heat olive oil in a pot over medium heat. Add the chopped onion and minced garlic, and sauté until translucent.
4. Add the black beans and vegetable broth. Bring to a boil, then reduce heat and simmer for 1 hour or until the beans are tender.
5. In a dry skillet, toast the black sesame seeds until fragrant.
6. Stir the sesame seeds into the soup.
7. Season with salt and pepper to taste and serve hot.

## 5. Mixed Nuts and Seeds Trail Mix

## Ingredients:

- 1/2 cup almonds
- 1/2 cup walnuts
- 1/4 cup pumpkin seeds
- 1/4 cup sunflower seeds
- 1/4 cup dried cranberries
- 1/4 cup dried goji berries

- 1/4 cup dark chocolate chips (optional)
- Pinch of salt

**Instructions:**

1. In a large bowl, combine all ingredients.
2. Mix well to ensure even distribution.
3. Store in an airtight container.
4. Serve as a snack whenever needed.

These recipes provide a variety of delicious ways to incorporate nuts and seeds into a postpartum diet, offering essential nutrients, energy, and support for lactation. By including these nutrient-dense foods in their daily meals, new mothers can enhance their recovery and overall well-being during the postpartum period.

# CONCLUSION

### The Journey of Postpartum Recovery

The postpartum period is a transformative journey that involves physical, emotional, and mental changes. It is a time when new mothers need to prioritize their health and well-being to recover from childbirth and adapt to the demands of caring for a newborn. The confinement period offers a structured approach to support this recovery, emphasizing the importance of rest, nutrition, and self-care. By following the practices and recipes outlined in this book, new mothers can enhance their healing process and build a strong foundation for their future health.

### Embracing the Confinement Period

Embracing the confinement period is about more than just adhering to traditional practices; it is about recognizing the value of self-care and nourishment during a critical time. The wisdom of traditional Chinese medicine, combined with modern adaptations, provides a comprehensive approach to postpartum recovery. By incorporating warming foods, protein-rich meals, iron-rich dishes, and herbal teas, new mothers can address their unique nutritional needs and promote overall well-being. The recipes and practices shared in this book are designed to be accessible, delicious, and supportive of the postpartum healing process.

### Long-Term Health Benefits

The benefits of a well-managed confinement period extend far beyond the immediate postpartum months. Proper nutrition, rest, and self-care during this time can have long-term positive effects on a mother's health. Enhanced immune function, balanced hormones, improved energy levels, and better mental health are just a few of the long-term benefits. By adopting healthy eating habits and self-care practices during confinement, new mothers can set the stage for a healthier and more balanced life.

## Encouraging a Balanced Diet Beyond Confinement

While the confinement period is crucial for recovery, maintaining a balanced diet and healthy lifestyle should be a lifelong commitment. The recipes and nutritional guidelines provided in this book can serve as a foundation for ongoing health and wellness. Embracing whole foods, balanced meals, and regular self-care practices can help new mothers sustain their energy, support their immune systems, and promote overall well-being long after the confinement period has ended.

In conclusion, the journey of postpartum recovery is an opportunity to nurture oneself and embrace the profound changes that come with motherhood. By prioritizing nutrition, rest, and self-care during the confinement period, new mothers can ensure a smoother recovery and lay the groundwork for long-term health and happiness. This book is a guide to navigating this transformative time with the support of nourishing recipes and traditional wisdom, empowering new mothers to take charge of their health and well-being.

# APPENDICES

**Common Ingredients in Confinement Recipes**

Many confinement recipes rely on specific ingredients that are known for their nutritional and medicinal properties. Here are some common ingredients used in confinement cooking:

1. **Ginger:** Known for its warming properties, ginger helps improve circulation and digestion.

2. **Red Dates (Jujubes):** Rich in vitamins and minerals, they help replenish blood and boost immunity.

3. **Goji Berries:** Packed with antioxidants, these berries support overall health and improve energy levels.

4. **Sesame Oil:** Used for its warming effect and high nutritional value.

5. **Chinese Herbs:** Various herbs like dang gui (angelica root) and wolfberries (goji berries) are used for their healing properties.

6. **Bone Broth:** Provides essential minerals and collagen to aid in healing and recovery.

7. **Leafy Greens:** Such as spinach and kale, for their high iron and vitamin content.

8. **Protein Sources:** Including chicken, pork, and fish, essential for muscle repair and recovery.

9. **Whole Grains:** Such as brown rice and millet, providing sustained energy.

**Glossary of Terms**

- **Confinement:** A traditional postpartum period where new mothers rest and follow specific dietary practices to aid recovery.

- **Traditional Chinese Medicine (TCM):** A holistic approach to health that includes herbal medicine, acupuncture, and dietary therapy.

- **Yin and Yang:** TCM concepts representing opposite but complementary forces in the body.

- **Qi:** The vital life force or energy that flows through the body.

- **Herbs:** Plants used for their medicinal properties.

## Where to Find Ingredients

Confinement ingredients can often be found at:

- **Asian Supermarkets:** Large chains often carry a wide variety of traditional herbs, spices, and foods used in confinement recipes.

- **Health Food Stores:** These stores often stock organic and specialty ingredients, including various nuts, seeds, and whole grains.

- **Online Retailers:** Websites like Amazon, Thrive Market, and specialty Asian food retailers can be a convenient source for hard-to-find ingredients.

- **Farmer's Markets:** Fresh, local produce and sometimes unique herbs and spices can be sourced here.

## Meal Planning and Preparation Tips

Proper planning and preparation can make the confinement period more manageable and enjoyable.

**Weekly Meal Plans** Create a weekly meal plan to ensure a balanced diet and avoid the stress of daily meal decisions. Here's a sample:

**Week 1:**

- **Breakfast:** Almond Milk Porridge, Yogurt with Goji Berries and Nuts
- **Lunch:** Sesame Oil Chicken with Red Dates, Stir-Fried Spinach with Garlic
- **Dinner:** Ginger and Vinegar Pig's Trotters, Chicken and Papaya Soup
- **Snacks:** Mixed Nuts and Seeds Trail Mix, Red Date and Longan Tea

**Week 2:**

- **Breakfast:** Chia Seed Pudding with Longan, Brown Rice Porridge with Red Dates
- **Lunch:** Beef and Spinach Stir-Fry, Sweet Potato and Carrot Mash
- **Dinner:** Fish and Papaya Soup, Turmeric Chicken Soup
- **Snacks:** Sunflower Seed and Goji Berry Snack Bars, Chinese Wolfberry Tea

**Shopping Lists** Create a comprehensive shopping list to streamline your grocery trips.

**Sample Shopping List:**

- Fresh Produce: Ginger, spinach, kale, sweet potatoes, carrots, papaya, bananas
- Proteins: Chicken, pork, fish, beef, eggs
- Grains: Brown rice, millet, oats
- Dairy and Alternatives: Almond milk, yogurt, cheese, chia seeds
- Nuts and Seeds: Almonds, walnuts, sesame seeds, sunflower seeds
- Herbs and Spices: Red dates, goji berries, Chinese herbs, turmeric, garlic

- Oils: Sesame oil, olive oil
- Sweeteners: Honey, maple syrup
- Miscellaneous: Coconut milk, almond butter

## Cooking Tips and Techniques

1. **Batch Cooking:** Prepare large portions of soups, broths, and grains to save time.

2. **Proper Storage:** Use airtight containers to keep ingredients fresh and prevent spoilage.

3. **Simple Techniques:** Focus on basic cooking methods like boiling, steaming, and stir-frying to retain nutrients.

4. **Flavor Enhancements:** Use herbs and spices to add flavor without relying on salt or sugar.

5. **Hydration:** Ensure soups and broths are well-hydrated to aid digestion and hydration.

By incorporating these meal planning and preparation tips, new mothers can make the confinement period more efficient and enjoyable, ensuring they receive the necessary nutrients to support their postpartum recovery.

Printed in Great Britain
by Amazon